Homemade Bath Salts

A Complete Beginner's Guide to Natural DIY Bath Salts you can Make Today

Jane Aniston

Introduction

What could be more relaxing than having a warm bath after a tough day at work? When you've had a long day there's nothing better than sitting back, relaxing and enjoying the scents and sensations that rejuvenating bath salts can provide.

In this book, you'll learn exactly how to make your very own bespoke bath salts at home, and all it takes is just a few simple ingredients. What's more, with a bit of creative thinking you can adjust the recipes to your liking, creating unique bath salt blends that yourself and your family can enjoy. Homemade bath salts also make great presents and I've even known people to go from making bath salts as a hobby to starting their own small businesses.

Have a good read through this book and you'll be on the right track to making your own bath salts in no time. The process is simple and you'll have tons of fun recreating the 35 unique recipes that are included.

Free of toxic nasties and packed with health promoting ingredients such as essential oils and herbs, these 35 bath salt recipes are not only fun to make, but will have you feeling both physically and mentally refreshed and rejuvenated in no time!

Thank you for downloading this book and good luck with your bath salt creations!

Jane Aniston

Table of contents

10. Spring Florals Bath Salts

11. Orange Rose Bath Salts

12. Green Tea Bath Salts

13. Baby Soft Skin Bath Salts

14. Summer Citrus Tea Bath Salts

15. Indian Garden Bath Salts

16. Sweet Chamomile Bath Salts

17. Wake Up Bath Salts

18. Sandalwood Spice Tea Bath Salts

19. Parisian Dreams Bath Salts

20. Earl Grey Bath Salts

21. Sweet Senses Bath Salts

22. Loving Feeling Bath Salts

23. Lavender Kisses Bath Salts

24. Orient Express Bath Salts

25. Sugar and Spice Bath Salts

26. Moulin Rouge Bath Salts

27. Flu Buster Bath Salts

28. Into the Woods Bath Salts

Chapter 6: Last Minute Tips and Reminders For Making Bath Salts

Conclusion

A message from the author, Jane Aniston

Chapter 1

Bath Salts And Their Benefits

Bath salts offer many benefits that go beyond the obvious of cleansing your body and smelling good. The right bath salt blend can help improve your skin texture as well as giving you a mental boost.

To some, bath salts may seem like a luxury item, but as you'll see in this book it really won't cost you much to give yourself the pampering you deserve. Here are just some of the amazing benefits you can enjoy once you get into the habit of using bath salts.

Smoother skin

Bath salts are great for smoothing out rough patches of skin. The secret? Little salt particles that exfoliate dead skin cells naturally. A small amount of finely ground sea salt rubbed gently on to damp skin can smoothen out the complexion and even promote healthy skin growth. Just remember to rub gently to avoid causing irritation to your skin.

Help detox your body

Salt contains minerals that easily get absorbed via the pores, and this in turn promotes healthy detoxification. If you want to do a detox without having to resort to some of the other potentially dangerous methods available, a good soak in salt water might just do the trick. Not only are you going to get clearer skin, but you'll also feel amazingly light after your warm salt bath. Bath salts with peppermint essential oils and olive oil are especially great for drawing out any impurities from your body.

Fights off stress and fatigue

Salt is also rich in minerals that can help fight off stress and fatigue. Calcium when absorbed through the pores prevents water retention while sodium plays an important role in keeping the balance of your body's lymphatic fluids. Salt also contains bromide to soothe sore and tired muscles, making salt baths the perfect post workout treat.

Make you look and feel younger

Salt's natural moisturizing properties will not only make you look younger, but you're also going to feel it as well! Regular bath salt use can restore your skin's moisture balance and plump it up over time. In just a few weeks of regular use, you may notice that the appearance of fine lines slowly fades and you'll emit a much healthier glow via your skin. What's great about using bath salts is that you don't need to buy expensive beauty products to get that youthful glow. Since you're using an all natural ingredient, there's no need to worry about any harmful chemical buildup in your system.

Affordable

Let's face it, looking young isn't exactly cheap! With most beauty treatments costing anywhere from $30 to $100 a pop, you can expect to spend a small fortune before you see any visible results. Bath salts are the perfect solution because you can enjoy all the beauty and health benefits for only a few dollars. You can easily erase a few years off of the appearance of your skin just by mixing your very own bath salt blends and using them when you soak in a warm bath. Now, doesn't that sound like a great plan?

Chapter 2

Basic Ingredients for Making your Own Bath Salts

One of the best things about making your own bath salts, aside from them being very affordable, is that they don't take much time or expertise to make, even when it comes to creating your very own blends. All you need are a few ingredients and some creative flair and voila! You have your very own blend of bath salts to make every bathing experience unique. If you're ready to get started on your bath salts journey, here's a list of the basic ingredients you'll need.

Salts

The first and most important ingredient you'll need is of course, salt. There's a wide array of different kinds of salts you can use to make your bath salts, depending on the benefits that you're aiming for. If you want a high mineral bath for example, sea salt is your best bet. On the other hand, if you want to create a more luxurious blend, pink Himalayan salt is the perfect choice.

Essential oils and carrier oils

One way to give your bath salts a unique personality is to add essential oils to them. Essential oils are natural plant extracts that offer healing benefits to the body. They don't just promote physical wellness, but also help improve your emotional state of mind. There are countless combinations that you can try, (and we'll talk more about some of them in the next chapter!), so don't be afraid to experiment with different blends. Carrier oils are oils that are used to dilute essential oils in. Since most essential oils come concentrated, you need to use a carrier oil to thin them out. Carrier oils can also offer healing and beautifying benefits, so always make sure to keep a high-quality carrier oil around. Great examples of carrier oils are good quality olive oil or jojoba oil.

Dried herbs

Adding dried herbs to your bath salts can give your creations that extra oomph. Not only do they offer additional healing benefits, but they also add a bit of artistic flair to the finished product. One drawback though that you'll need to watch out for is the mess that these herbal additions will leave in the tub after you finish your bath!

Baking soda

Baking soda mixed with salt can help detoxify your body. It can also help soothe itchiness caused by allergic reactions. Baking soda softens hard water without any need for expensive bath bombs.

Citric acid

Although citric acid is more commonly used in bath bomb making, it can add an interesting twist to your bath salts blend. The combination of salt and citric acid creates a fizzing effect that doesn't just soften skin, but also helps release the aroma of your bath salts into the air. It creates an aromatic bath experience that will be both uplifting and refreshing.

Powdered milk

Not one of the usual ingredients you'll see on most bath salt recipes, but it is an ingredient that can make a big difference in your bathing routine. Milk contains lactic acid that can help exfoliate dead skin cells and promote healthy skin cell regeneration, so adding a scoop or two to your bath salt blend can do wonders for your skin. You can use just about any powdered milk you have; just be sure you take note of the best before date!

Food colorant

You can create colorful bath salts by adding a teeny bit of food colorant into the mix. Food colorant is a safe and inexpensive way to color your batch of bath salts without any fear that it will stain your skin or your tub. Bath salt aficionados recommend liquid food color because they only add a tinge of color to your bath salts.

Chapter 3

Top 10 Essential Oils for Bath Salts

As mentioned earlier, the essential oil you decide to use will play a big part in giving your bath salts their healing and rejuvenating properties. Essential oils not only add scent to your bath salt creations, but they also pack in a number of health and wellness benefits. If you have yet to start building up your essential oils collection, then here's a list of the top 10 oils you should have have in your home. Warning: be careful not to get the oils on your clothing as some may be hard to remove!

Lavender

As one of the most well-loved and popular essential oils available, lavender should definitely be first on the list! Its relaxing and calming properties can help reduce stress and set your body up for a restful night sleep.

Chamomile

Although chamomile is best known for it's use as a herbal tea, this essential oil shares similar properties to lavender, but has a more subtle scent. Just add a few drops into your bath salts and you're sure to feel calm and relaxed.

Peppermint

Peppermint, on the other hand, can help increase mental alertness and promote mental stimulation. Use this to wake yourself up in the morning if you think you're likely to have a grueling and mentally challenging day ahead. Peppermint is also one of the few oils that are actually safe to ingest.

Oregano

Oregano is known for its potent antibacterial properties, making it the perfect essential oil for those who's skin is prone to breakouts. Just add a few drops into your bath salts to help promote clear skin. In addition, it is also the perfect choice whenever you feel under the weather as it can help fight off colds and similar illnesses.

Frankincense

Frankincense isn't just great for relaxation, but when applied topically, it can also help heal minor cuts and soothe insect bites. Frankincense is an essential oil that has been used for centuries. Some say this essential oil can also help increase spiritual awareness.

Tea tree

Are you looking for an all-natural solution to treat skin problems caused by fungal infections? Then add a few drops of tea tree essential oil into your bath salts and say goodbye to athlete's foot forever! It also acts as a great option for combatting acne, so if you have problems with acne, this might just be the solution you are looking for.

Calendula

Calendula, also known as marigold is great for those who have sensitive skin. It's so gentle and mild that many people use it to treat psoriasis. You can also apply a few drops to any affected areas if you want to reduce the appearance of acne scars and dark marks.

Grapefruit

Need an instant perk me up to get rid of tiredness? Then the scent of grapefruit might just do the trick! Although grapefruit essential oil acts as a natural antiseptic that can cleanse and exfoliate the skin, it can also cause skin irritation to those with sensitive skin. Make sure to mix grapefruit essential oil with a carrier oil like olive oil or jojoba oil before use if you want to apply it topically.

Lemon

Not to be outdone by its citrus relative, lemon can also work wonders on cleansing and exfoliating skin. Its smoothing and whitening properties can help fade acne scars with continued use. For those who are feeling stressed or overwhelmed, this oil can also be used to uplift mood and increase concentration.

Eucalyptus

If you need a little of help unblocking nasal congestion or clogged sinuses, then eucalyptus essential oil is perfect for boosting your immune system. Its antibacterial properties can also help save you from getting colds come the winter season. Be sure to dilute eucalyptus essential oil with a carrier oil as it can be a little too strong for those with sensitive skin.

Chapter 4

Insider Tips On Creating Your Own Bath Salts

Creating your own bath salts can be quite an experience. Not only do you get to create something amazingly relaxing, you also have the opportunity to learn more about how different ingredients can offer different scents and sensations.

It doesn't matter where you got your inspiration from, the important thing is that you've taken that first step to making your own bath salts which will be a lot of fun and allow you to create top-quality products.

However, there are some things you should be aware of before you begin. So before you grab that mixing bowl, here are a few insider tips to get you off to a good start and help you avoid any problems further down the road.

Prep your workspace

The first thing you need to do before you get started on your bath salts is to prep your workspace. Making your own bath salts at home can get quite messy, so make sure that you have prepared a dedicated space for it which will be easy to clean up when you've finished. Working in the kitchen is perfectly fine, but if you're going to turn it into a habit, you might want to look around your home for a small area you can dedicate to bath salts creation, space permitting of course.

Source your ingredients from a reliable supplier

Most of the ingredients needed to make your own homemade bath salts can easily be bought from local stores. However, if you're looking for an ingredient that can't be easily purchased in your area, you can always find a reliable supplier online with a little searching. When sourcing ingredients, make sure to choose a supplier that is known first and foremost for their quality, and not just the quantity of product they are offering. Don't be fooled by a cheap price tag if you're not sure about the quality of the product.

Be aware of your allergies

Just because an ingredient is considered all-natural or organic doesn't mean that it's guaranteed to be 100%

safe for you. It may work wonders for others, but there is the odd chance that for you it could cause an allergic reaction. So before you get started on any homemade bath salt batches, make sure that the ingredients you're going to use are safe for you. Try to figure out which (if any) of the common ingredients may cause skin irritation. If you're going to work with an unfamiliar ingredient, test it first on your wrist to see if it causes a negative reaction. This way, you don't end up harming your skin.

Always store homemade bath salts in appropriate containers

Once you've made a fresh batch of DIY bath salts, it's critical that you store it in an appropriate container. Look for containers with airtight lids so your product won't be exposed to air, humidity, germs, and bacteria. Although not essential, glass containers are a good option as glass is inert, meaning no chemicals will be able to leach into your bath salts.

Don't get too hung up on following the recipes to the letter

The amounts of the ingredients you'll need may sometimes seem a little vague, but don't get too hung up on being exact; just follow the instructions as best you can to begin with. Making your own bath salts is a lot like cooking; over time you'll get used to the recipes and will be able to adjust them to suit your own needs and preferences.

Now that you're well prepared, let's get started on the recipes! Good luck!

Chapter 5

Homemade Bath Salt Recipes

1. Peppermint Fresh Bath Salts

Ingredients:

- 1 cup sea salt

- 1 cup Epsom salt

- ½ teaspoon peppermint essential oil

- ½ teaspoon Olive oil

- 2 tablespoons dried peppermint leaves, chopped finely

- 1-2 drops of green food color

Instructions:

1. Measure ingredients.

2. Combine sea salt and Epsom salt in a bowl.

3. Slowly add peppermint oil and olive oil. Be sure to mix all ingredients thoroughly.

4. Store bath salts in a glass jar with cover.

5. To use: Sprinkle a couple of tablespoons of bath salts into warm bath water and enjoy!

2. Happy Days Bath Salts

Ingredients:

- 1 cup Epsom salt

- 1 cup baking soda

- 2 tablespoon liquid glycerin

- ½ teaspoon bergamot essential oil

- ½ teaspoon clary Sage essential oil

- ½ teaspoon sunflower oil

Instructions:

1. Measure ingredients.

2. Combine Epsom salt and baking soda together.

3. Add the liquid glycerin and make sure to mix well with the dry ingredients.

4. Add clary sage, bergamot, and sunflower oils.

5. Pour bath salts into a glass container with an airtight lid.

6. To use: Add 2 tablespoons of bath salts to warm bath water and enjoy!

3. Baby Fresh Bath Salts

Ingredients:

- 1 cup Epsom salts
- ½ cup citric acid
- ½ cup baking soda
- 1 teaspoon calendula essential oil
- 1 teaspoon jasmine essential oil
- 1-2 drops of blue food color

Instructions:

1. Mix Epsom salts and baking soda in a small bowl.

2. Add essential oils and food color, one drop at a time, until you get your desired scent and color. Mix well.

3. Add citric acid and stir mixture.

4. Store in glass jars with airtight lids.

5. To use: Add a couple of tablespoons to bath water and enjoy!

4. Blue Lagoon Bath Salts

Ingredients:

- 1 cup sea salt
- 1 cup powdered milk
- 1 teaspoon eucalyptus essential oil
- 1 teaspoon olive oil
- Drops of blue food color

Instructions:

1. Measure ingredients.

2. Combine salt and powdered milk in a bowl.

3. Add eucalyptus oil and olive oil and mix well.

4. Add blue food color, one drop at a time, until you get the color you want.

5. Store in airtight glass containers.

6. To use: Add 2 teaspoons of bath salts to bath water for a moisturizing soak and enjoy!

5. Italian Breeze Bath Salts

Ingredients:

- 1 cup sea salt

- 1 cup Epsom salt

- ¼ teaspoon basil essential oil

- ¼ teaspoon oregano essential oil

- ½ teaspoon olive oil

- 2 tablespoons dried basil leaves, chopped finely

- 1-2 drops of green food color

Instructions:

1. Measure ingredients.

2. Combine sea salt and Epsom salt in a bowl.

3. Slowly add basil oil and oregano oil with the olive oil. Be sure to spread the oils and mix all ingredients thoroughly.

4. Add basil leaves and green food color to the salt.

5. Store bath salts in a glass jar with cover.

6. To use: Sprinkle a couple of tablespoons of bath salts into warm bath water and enjoy!

6. Refresher Bath Salts

Ingredients:

- 1 cup Epsom salt
- 1 cup baking soda
- 2 tablespoon liquid glycerin
- 1 teaspoon eucalyptus essential oil
- ½ teaspoon geranium essential oil
- ½ teaspoon sweet almond oil

Instructions:

1. Measure ingredients.
2. Combine Epsom salt and baking soda together.
3. Add the liquid glycerin and make sure to mix well with the dry ingredients.
4. Add the eucalyptus essential oil, geranium essential oil, and sweet almond oil.
5. Pour bath salts into a glass container with an airtight lid.

6. To use: Add 2 tablespoons of bath salts to warm bath water and enjoy!

7. Confidence Booster Bath Salts

Ingredients:

- 1 cup Epsom salts
- ½ cup citric acid
- ½ cup baking soda
- 1 teaspoon orange essential oil
- 1 teaspoon rosemary essential oil
- 1-2 drops of red and yellow food color

Instructions:

1. Mix Epsom salts and baking soda in a small bowl.

2. Add essential oils and food color, one drop at a time, until you get your desired scent and color. Mix well.

3. Add citric acid and stir mixture.

4. Store in glass jars with airtight lids.

5. To use: Add a couple of tablespoons to bath water and enjoy!

8. Milky Rose Bath Salts

Ingredients:

- 1 cup sea salt

- 1 cup powdered milk

- 1 teaspoon rose essential oil

- 1 teaspoon sunflower oil

- Drops of red food color

Instructions:

1. Measure ingredients.

2. Combine salt and powdered milk in a bowl.

3. Add rose essential oil and sunflower oil and mix well.

4. Add red food color, one drop at a time, until you get the color you want.

5. Store in airtight glass containers.

6. To use: Add 2 teaspoons of bath salts to bath water for a moisturizing soak and enjoy!

9. Sweet Dreams Bath Salts

Ingredients:

- 1 cup sea salt

- 1 cup Epsom salt

- ½ teaspoon lavender essential oil

- ½ teaspoon evening primrose oil

- 2 tablespoons dried lavender flowers, chopped finely

Instructions:

1. Measure ingredients.

2. Combine sea salt and Epsom salt in a bowl.

3. Slowly add lavender essential oil and evening primrose oil. Be sure to spread the oils and mix all ingredients thoroughly.

4. Add dried lavender to the mix and stir well.

5. Store bath salts in a glass jar with cover.

6. To use: Sprinkle a couple of tablespoons of bath salts into warm bath water and enjoy!

10. Spring Florals Bath Salts

Ingredients:

- 1 cup Epsom salt
- 1 cup baking soda
- 2 tablespoon liquid glycerin
- ½ teaspoon rose essential oil
- ½ lavender essential oil
- ½ teaspoon sunflower oil
- 1 teaspoon dried lavender, chopped

Instructions:

1. Measure ingredients.
2. Combine Epsom salt and baking soda together.
3. Add the liquid glycerin and make sure to mix well with the dry ingredients.
4. Add the rose essential oil, lavender essential oil, and sunflower oil.
5. Add dried lavender to the mix and stir well.

6. Pour bath salts into a glass container with an airtight lid.

7. To use: Add 2 tablespoons of bath salts to warm bath water and enjoy!

11. Orange Rose Bath Salts

Ingredients:

- 1 cup Epsom salts
- ½ cup citric acid
- ½ cup baking soda
- 1 teaspoon rose essential oil
- 1 teaspoon orange essential oil
- 1-2 drops of red and yellow food color

Instructions:

1. Mix Epsom salts and baking soda in a small bowl.

2. Add essential oils and food color, one drop at a time, until you get your desired scent and color. Mix well.

3. Add citric acid and stir mixture.

4. Store in glass jars with airtight lids.

5. To use: Add a couple of tablespoons to bath water and enjoy!

12. Green Tea Bath Salts

Ingredients:

- 1 cup sea salt

- 1 cup powdered milk

- 1 teaspoon peppermint essential oil

- 1 teaspoon sweet almond oil

- 1 teaspoon dried green tea

- Drops of green food color

Instructions:

1. Measure ingredients.

2. Combine salt and powdered milk in a bowl.

3. Add peppermint essential oil and sweet almond oil and mix well.

4. Add green food color, one drop at a time, until you get the color you want.

5. Add dried green tea leaves and stir well.

6. Store in airtight glass containers.

7. To use: Add 2 teaspoons of bath salts to bath water for a moisturizing soak and enjoy!

13. Baby Soft Skin Bath Salts

Ingredients:

- 1 cup sea salt

- 1 cup Epsom salt

- ½ teaspoon Ylang Ylang essential oil

- ¼ teaspoon sunflower oil

- ¼ teaspoon jojoba oil

- 1 drop of red food color

Instructions:

1. Measure ingredients.

2. Combine sea salt and Epsom salt in a bowl.

3. Slowly add Ylang Ylang essential oil, sunflower oil and jojoba oil. Be sure to spread the oils and mix all ingredients thoroughly.

4. Add 1 drop of red food color to add a pink tinge to the salts.

5. Store bath salts in a glass jar with cover.

6. To use: Sprinkle a couple of tablespoons of bath salts into warm bath water and enjoy!

14. Summer Citrus Tea Bath Salts

Ingredients:

- 1 cup Epsom salt
- 1 cup baking soda
- 2 tablespoon liquid glycerin
- ½ teaspoon orange essential oil
- ½ teaspoon grapefruit essential oil
- ½ teaspoon sweet almond oil

Instructions:

1. Measure ingredients.

2. Combine Epsom salt and baking soda together.

3. Add the liquid glycerin and make sure to mix well with the dry ingredients.

4. Add the orange essential oil, grapefruit essential oil, and sweet almond oil and stir well.

5. Pour bath salts into a glass container with an airtight lid.

6. To use: Add 2 tablespoons of bath salts to warm bath water and enjoy!

15. Indian Garden Bath Salts

Ingredients:

- 1 cup Epsom salts
- ½ cup citric acid
- ½ cup baking soda
- 1 teaspoon frankincense essential oil
- 1 teaspoon Ylang Ylang essential
- 1 teaspoon jasmine essential oil
- 1-2 drops of red food color

Instructions:

1. Mix Epsom salts and baking soda in a small bowl.

2. Add essential oils and food color, one drop at a time, until you get your desired scent and color. Mix well.

3. Add citric acid and stir mixture.

4. Store in glass jars with airtight lids.

5. To use: Add a couple of tablespoons to bath water and enjoy!

16. Sweet Chamomile Bath Salts

Ingredients:

- 1 cup sea salt

- 1 cup powdered milk

- 1 teaspoon chamomile essential oil

- 1 teaspoon sweet almond oil

- 1 teaspoon dried chamomile tea

- Drops of yellow food color

Instructions:

1. Measure ingredients.

2. Combine salt and powdered milk in a bowl.

3. Add chamomile essential oil and sweet almond oil and mix well.

4. Add yellow food color, one drop at a time, until you get the color you want.

5. Sprinkle dried chamomile tealeaves and stir well.

6. Store in airtight glass containers.

7. To use: Add 2 teaspoons of bath salts to bath water for a moisturizing soak and enjoy!

17. Wake Up Bath Salts

Ingredients:

- 1 cup sea salt

- 1 cup Epsom salt

- ½ teaspoon peppermint essential oil

- ¼ teaspoon rosemary essential oil

- ½ teaspoon jojoba oil

- 2 tablespoons dried rosemary sprigs, chopped finely

Instructions:

1. Measure ingredients.

2. Combine sea salt and Epsom salt in a bowl.

3. Slowly add peppermint oil, rosemary oil and jojoba oil. Be sure to spread the oils and mix all ingredients thoroughly.

4. Add dried rosemary sprigs and stir well.

5. Store bath salts in a glass jar with cover.

6. To use: Sprinkle a couple of tablespoons of bath salts into warm bath water and enjoy!

18. Sandalwood Spice Tea Bath Salts

Ingredients:

- 1 cup Epsom salt

- 1 cup baking soda

- 2 tablespoon liquid glycerin

- 1 teaspoon sandalwood essential oil

- ½ teaspoon sweet almond oil

Instructions:

1. Measure ingredients.

2. Combine Epsom salt and baking soda together.

3. Add the liquid glycerin and make sure to mix well with the dry ingredients.

4. Add the sandalwood essential oil and sweet almond oil.

5. Pour bath salts into a glass container with an airtight lid.

6. To use: Add 2 tablespoons of bath salts to warm bath water and enjoy!

19. Parisian Dreams Bath Salts

Ingredients:

- 1 cup Epsom salts
- ½ cup citric acid
- ½ cup baking soda
- 1 teaspoon bergamot essential oil
- 1 teaspoon chamomile essential oil
- 1-2 drops of yellow food color

Instructions:

1. Mix Epsom salts and baking soda in a small bowl.

2. Add essential oils and food color, one drop at a time, until you get your desired scent and color. Mix well.

3. Add citric acid and stir mixture.

4. Store in glass jars with airtight lids.

5. To use: Add a couple of tablespoons to bath water and enjoy!

20. Earl Grey Bath Salts

Ingredients:

- 1 cup sea salt
- 1 cup powdered milk
- 1 teaspoon bergamot essential oil
- 1 teaspoon Olive oil
- 1 teaspoon dried earl grey leaves
- Drops of green food color

Instructions:

1. Measure ingredients.
2. Combine salt and powdered milk in a bowl.
3. Add bergamot essential oil and olive oil and mix well.
4. Add green food color, one drop at a time, until you get the color you want.
5. Add dried earl grey tea leaves and stir well.
6. Store in airtight glass containers.

7. To use: Add 2 teaspoons of bath salts to bath water for a moisturizing soak and enjoy!

21. Sweet Senses Bath Salts

Ingredients:

- 1 cup sea salt
- 1 cup Epsom salt
- ¼ teaspoon vanilla essential oil
- ½ teaspoon rose essential oil
- ½ teaspoon sunflower oil
- 2 tablespoons dried rose petals, chopped finely
- 2 drops of red food color

Instructions:

1. Measure ingredients.
2. Combine sea salt and Epsom salt in a bowl.
3. Slowly add vanilla essential oil, rose essential oil, and sunflower oil. Be sure to spread the oils and mix all ingredients thoroughly.
4. Add dried rose petals and stir well.
5. Store bath salts in a glass jar with cover.

6. To use: Sprinkle a couple of tablespoons of bath salts into warm bath water and enjoy!

22. Loving Feeling Bath Salts

Ingredients:

- 1 cup Epsom salt
- 1 cup baking soda
- 2 tablespoon liquid glycerin
- 1 teaspoon Ylang Ylang essential oil
- 1 teaspoon clary sage essential oil
- ½ teaspoon jojoba oil

Instructions:

1. Measure ingredients.

2. Combine Epsom salt and baking soda together.

3. Add the liquid glycerin and make sure to mix well with the dry ingredients.

4. Add the Ylang Ylang essential oil, clary sage essential oil, and jojoba oil.

5. Pour bath salts into a glass container with an airtight lid.

6. To use: Add 2 tablespoons of bath salts to warm bath water and enjoy!

23. Lavender Kisses Bath Salts

Ingredients:

- 1 cup Epsom salts
- ½ cup citric acid
- ½ cup baking soda
- 1 teaspoon lavender essential oil
- 1 teaspoon clary sage essential oil
- 1-2 drops of blue food color

Instructions:

1. Mix Epsom salts and baking soda in a small bowl.

2. Add essential oils and food color, one drop at a time, until you get your desired scent and color. Mix well.

3. Add citric acid and stir mixture.

4. Store in glass jars with airtight lids.

5. To use: Add a couple of tablespoons to bath water and enjoy!

24. Orient Express Bath Salts

Ingredients:

- 1 cup sea salt

- 1 cup Epsom salt

- ¼ teaspoon patchouli essential oil

- ¼ teaspoon orange essential oil

- ½ teaspoon coconut oil

- 2 drops of yellow food color

Instructions:

1. Measure ingredients.

2. Combine sea salt and Epsom salt in a bowl.

3. Slowly add patchouli essential oil, orange essential oil, and coconut oil. Be sure to spread the oils and mix all ingredients thoroughly.

4. Add yellow food color and stir well.

5. Store bath salts in a glass jar with cover.

6. To use: Sprinkle a couple of tablespoons of bath salts into warm bath water and enjoy!

25. Sugar and Spice Bath Salts

Ingredients:

- 1 cup Epsom salt

- 1 cup baking soda

- 2 tablespoon liquid glycerin

- 1/2 teaspoon orange essential oil

- ¼ teaspoon cinnamon essential oil

- ¼ teaspoon ginger essential oil

- ½ teaspoon sweet almond oil

Instructions:

1. Measure ingredients.

2. Combine Epsom salt and baking soda together.

3. Add the liquid glycerin and make sure to mix well with the dry ingredients.

4. Add orange essential oil, cinnamon essential oil, ginger essential oil, and sweet almond oil.

5. Pour bath salts into a glass container with an airtight lid.

6. To use: Add 2 tablespoons of bath salts to warm bath water and enjoy!

26. Moulin Rouge Bath Salts

Ingredients:

- 1 cup Epsom salts
- ½ cup citric acid
- ½ cup baking soda
- 1 teaspoon rose essential oil
- 1 teaspoon sandalwood essential oil
- ½ teaspoon orange essential oil
- 1-2 drops of red food color

Instructions:

1. Mix Epsom salts and baking soda in a small bowl.

2. Add essential oils and food color, one drop at a time, until you get your desired scent and color. Mix well.

3. Add citric acid and stir mixture.

4. Store in glass jars with airtight lids.

5. To use: Add a couple of tablespoons to bath water and enjoy!

27. Flu Buster Bath Salts

Ingredients:

- 1 cup sea salt

- 1 cup Epsom salt

- ½ teaspoon lemon essential oil

- ¼ teaspoon eucalyptus essential oil

- ½ teaspoon coconut oil

- 2 tablespoons dried peppermint leaves, chopped finely

- 2 drops of blue food color

Instructions:

1. Measure ingredients.

2. Combine sea salt and Epsom salt in a bowl.

3. Slowly add lemon essential oil, eucalyptus essential oil and coconut oil. Be sure to spread the oils and mix all ingredients thoroughly.

4. Add dried peppermint leaves and stir well.

5. Store bath salts in a glass jar with cover.

6. To use: Sprinkle a couple of tablespoons of bath salts into warm bath water and enjoy!

28. Into the Woods Bath Salts

Ingredients:

- 1 cup Epsom salt

- 1 cup baking soda

- 2 tablespoon liquid glycerin

- 1 teaspoon frankincense essential oil

- 1 teaspoon grapefruit essential oil

- 1 teaspoon olive oil

Instructions:

1. Measure ingredients.

2. Combine Epsom salt and baking soda together.

3. Add the liquid glycerin and make sure to mix well with the dry ingredients.

4. Add the frankincense essential oil, grapefruit essential oil, and olive oil.

5. Pour bath salts into a glass container with an airtight lid.

6. To use: Add 2 tablespoons of bath salts to warm bath water and enjoy!

29. Perk me Up Bath Salts

Ingredients:

- 1 cup Epsom salts
- ½ cup citric acid
- ½ cup baking soda
- 1 teaspoon frankincense essential oil
- 1 teaspoon lemon essential oil
- ½ teaspoon jasmine essential oil
- 1-2 drops of yellow food color

Instructions:

1. Mix Epsom salts and baking soda in a small bowl.

2. Add essential oils and food color, one drop at a time, until you get your desired scent and color. Mix well.

3. Add citric acid and stir mixture.

4. Store in glass jars with airtight lids.

5. To use: Add a couple of tablespoons to bath water and enjoy!

30. Clean and Clear Bath Salts

Ingredients:

- 1 cup sea salt

- 1 cup Epsom salt

- ½ teaspoon tea tree essential oil

- ¼ teaspoon sandalwood essential oil

- ½ teaspoon olive oil

Instructions:

1. Measure ingredients.

2. Combine sea salt and Epsom salt in a bowl.

3. Slowly add tea tree essential oil, sandalwood essential oil and olive oil. Be sure to spread the oils and mix all ingredients thoroughly.

4. Store bath salts in a glass jar with cover.

5. To use: Sprinkle a couple of tablespoons of bath salts into warm bath water and enjoy!

31. Sweet Grapefruit Bath Salts

Ingredients:

- 1 cup Epsom salt

- 1 cup baking soda

- 2 tablespoon liquid glycerin

- 1 teaspoon grapefruit essential oil

- ½ teaspoon cypress essential oil

- ½ teaspoon sweet almond oil

Instructions:

1. Measure ingredients.

2. Combine Epsom salt and baking soda together.

3. Add the liquid glycerin and make sure to mix well with the dry ingredients.

4. Add the grapefruit essential oil, cypress essential oil, and sweet almond oil.

5. Pour bath salts into a glass container with an airtight lid.

6. To use: Add 2 tablespoons of bath salts to warm bath water and enjoy!

32. Morning Energy Bath Salts

Ingredients:

- 1 cup Epsom salts
- ½ cup citric acid
- ½ cup baking soda
- 1 teaspoon basil essential oil
- 1 teaspoon grapefruit essential oil
- 1-2 drops of green food color

Instructions:

1. Mix Epsom salts and baking soda in a small bowl.

2. Add essential oils and food color, one drop at a time, until you get your desired scent and color. Mix well.

3. Add citric acid and stir mixture.

4. Store in glass jars with airtight lids.

5. To use: Add a couple of tablespoons to bath water and enjoy!

33. Energy Boost Bath Salts

Ingredients:

- 1 cup sea salt
- 1 cup Epsom salt
- ½ teaspoon marjoram essential oil
- ¼ teaspoon ginger essential oil
- ½ teaspoon grapeseed oil
- 2 drops of yellow food color

Instructions:

1. Measure ingredients.

2. Combine sea salt and Epsom salt in a bowl.

3. Slowly add marjoram essential oil, ginger essential oil, and grapeseed oil. Be sure to spread the oils and mix all ingredients thoroughly.

4. Add yellow food color for a light tinge of sunshine.

5. Store bath salts in a glass jar with cover.

6. To use: Sprinkle a couple of tablespoons of bath salts into warm bath water and enjoy!

34. Chamomile Tea Bath Salts

Ingredients:

- 1 cup Epsom salt
- 1 cup baking soda
- 2 tablespoon liquid glycerin
- 1 teaspoon Chamomile essential oil
- ½ teaspoon sunflower oil

Instructions:

1. Measure ingredients.
2. Combine Epsom salt and baking soda together.
3. Add the liquid glycerin and make sure to mix well with the dry ingredients.
4. Add the chamomile essential oil and sunflower oil.
5. Pour bath salts into a glass container with an airtight lid.
6. To use: Add 2 tablespoons of bath salts to warm bath water and enjoy!

35. Soulmates Bath Salts

Ingredients:

- 1 cup Epsom salts
- ½ cup citric acid
- ½ cup baking soda
- 1 teaspoon grapefruit essential oil
- 1 teaspoon ginger essential oil
- 1-2 drops of red food color

Instructions:

1. Mix Epsom salts and baking soda in a small bowl.

2. Add essential oils and food color, one drop at a time, until you get your desired scent and color. Mix well.

3. Add citric acid and stir mixture.

4. Store in glass jars with airtight lids.

5. To use: Add a couple of tablespoons to bath water and enjoy!

Chapter 6

Last Minute Tips and Reminders

For Making Bath Salts

Even though making bath salts is not exactly rocket science, there are a few things that you need to remember in order to make sure things go smoothly. Whether you're making bath salts for personal use or for gifts, here are some last minute tips and reminders you might want to keep in mind.

Do a patch test with essential oils before use

Some essential oils have a tendency to cause irritation to sensitive skin so if you're not sure about a certain blend, it's probably best that you do a patch test first. Apply a drop of your chosen essential oil to a hidden area of your skin, preferably somewhere on the inside of your elbow. If you don't see any sign of irritation on the area within 24 hours, feel free to use that essential oil in your bath salts blend.

Allow the mixture to dry completely

To avoid getting rock hard bath salts, make sure that you allow the mixture to dry or sit overnight before storing it in your containers. By allowing the salts to dry completely, you won't have to deal with the drama of having lumpy bath salts. Bath salt recipes with glycerin are especially prone to lumpiness so make sure you give those bath salts enough time to cure before storing.

Store salts in non-metallic containers

Avoid storing bath salts in metallic containers if you don't want to compromise their quality over time. Salts and citric acid have a tendency to corrode metals so it's best to store your bath salts in glass or plastic containers. The great thing about storing bath salts in a glass container is it is more likely to maintain the integrity of the scents and essential oils that you used. It is also a great way to recycle those glass containers you have lying around the house. Do n't forget to get creative when decorating any containers you plan to give away as gifts in order to give that added flair!

Add a small scooper into your container

For convenience's sake, make sure that you add a small scooper into your bath salts container so that you don't need to pour the container and end up putting too much or too little in your bath. Having a small plastic or wooden scooper will also help if you need to loosen up salt clumps. A scooper is a must have if your bathroom is prone to high humidity because too much water vapor in the air will only make your bath salts clump together.

Shake the jar regularly

To make scooping out bath salts even easier, make sure that you shake your bath salts container regularly. A few shakes every now and then should be enough to keep your bath salts lump free and ready for use.

Conclusion

I hope that you now feel you have all the information you need in order to get started on making your very own bath salts. There's a whole world of different ingredients and scents to try so this is a great opportunity for you to explore your creative side.

As you already know by now, it doesn't take much in terms of either effort or money to make your very own bespoke bath products. As long as you follow the instructions carefully and use only the best ingredients, you'll be enjoying long luxurious baths which offer both healing and relaxing properties. Don't forget to have fun when making your very first batch of bath salts, and good luck!

A message from the author, Jane Aniston

Finally, if you enjoyed this book, **please** take the time to post a review on Amazon. It will only take a couple of minutes and I'd be extremely grateful for your support.

Jane Aniston

FREE BONUS!: Preview Of "Homemade Makeup - A Complete Beginner's Guide to Natural DIY Cosmetics You Can Make Today" - Includes 28 Organic Makeup Recipes!'

If you enjoyed this book, I have a little bonus for you; a preview of one of my other books "Homemade Makeup - A Complete Beginner's Guide to Natural DIY Cosmetics You Can Make Today", which exposes the secrets of the hidden toxins lurking in your store-bought cosmetics! This book also includes 28 simple and enjoyable organic makeup recipes that you can make at home today. Give yourself a glamorous look without exposing yourself to potentially harmful chemical nasties! Enjoy!

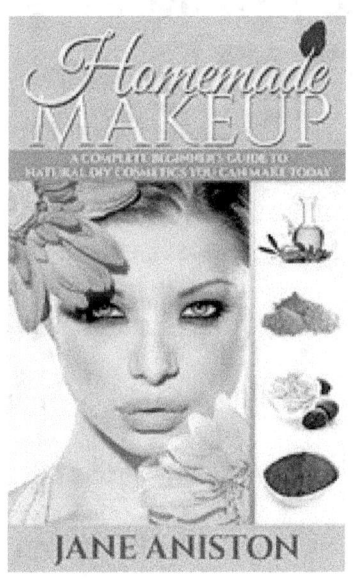

Chapter 1: Why you should stop using store-bought makeup and start making your own at home!

Makeup is something most women simply can't live without. Some women, in their search for beauty, have even gone as far getting permanent cosmetics tattooed on their faces (permanent eyebrows, for example). Personally, I see nothing wrong with wanting to look your best, but at the end of the day, one question we need to ask ourselves is: "What exactly are the ingredients in my beauty products?"

With almost all cosmetics containing numerous chemical ingredients, it can be a bit unsettling to think about the potential long-term effects these ingredients could be having on our bodies. Behind the glamour of the cosmetics industry, there's always the danger that the products we think are safe to put on our skin, might in actuality not be as safe as we think.

After studying the cosmetics industry, the truth is that these products have some of the largest mark-ups of any you're likely to find on the high street or in the mall! Your favorite face cream that cost you $80 may well have only cost as little as $2 to make, while that trendy lipstick you paid $30 of your hard-earned money for may actually only have a monetary value of $0.75! If you've bought thousands of dollars worth of cosmetics over the years, this realization can be pretty depressing. It doesn't feel good to know that all this time we've been duped by the cosmetics industry via slick marketing campaigns, while they made massive profits out of us unsuspecting consumers.

This is certainly something I've been a victim of. In the past, one of the things I would regularly spend money on was a good (and very expensive!) lipstick. Whenever I was having a bad day, I would head down to my favorite store and treat myself to a new shade. My friends would easily be able to tell if I was having a good year or not by the number of lipsticks I had in my collection! In hindsight, knowing what I know now, I feel a real sense of regret that I didn't get around to making my own cosmetics earlier. If I had of done, my bank balance certainly would have been a little healthier, and that money could have been better put to use.

The thing about the cosmetics industry is that even if you have a suspicion you're being ripped-off, it just feels that buying these products is something you *have to do*. I know a lot of women who would gladly fork over an inordinate amount of money for an excellent foundation! Why? Because you simply can't put a price on the confidence that looking your best can give you. The marketing used to sell cosmetic products has preyed on the insecurities of women for far too long. We are constantly bombarded with the message that if you want to feel good about yourself you need to look like a cover model; the implication being that the only way you'll be able to do that is to use their (expensive!) cosmetics. It's even gotten to the point where some women consider certain brands of makeup to be status symbols, much like they may do with a pair of expensive shoes or a designer handbag.

Am I immune to the marketing hype surrounding cosmetics? Honestly, no. I confess that even after learning the heartbreaking truth about the beauty industry I still get excited when I'm in the store browsing the makeup department. I still look at each lipstick color and eye shadow shade and imagine how I would incorporate them to achieve all sorts of glamorous looks. The only difference now is I don't purchase anywhere near as many products as I used to. These days I usually just look around in search of color inspiration, make a mental note and then create my own cosmetics at home. If you're thinking that the only reason I do this is to save a few dollars, you're wrong. Unfortunately there's more to it than that.

Harmful Ingredients Abound!

One of the sad realities when it comes to cosmetics is that the vast majority contain toxic ingredients. Even makeup products labeled as "all-natural" often times contain ingredients that may increase susceptibility to skin allergies, cancer, infertility and reproductive problems. If you're not sure about which ingredients you'd be best to avoid, here's a list of chemical nasties which are often used in cosmetics. Considering that human skin absorbs almost 60% of what is applied to it, this list will make you think twice next time you're about to splurge on expensive cosmetics.

- **Coal Tar** – Although already banned in the EU and Southeast Asia, there are still some products being sold in the US that contain this carcinogen. It's often found in treatments for dry skin as well as in anti-dandruff shampoos. Coal tar is also known as FD&C Red No.6.

- **Ethoxylated surfactants and 1,4-dioxane** – Created when carcinogenic ethylene oxide is added to a cocktail of other chemicals. This nasty toxin is found in some cosmetics, and unfortunately, is commonly found in baby washes being sold in the US. As a general rule, if you want to err on the safe side, avoid ingredients that contain the syllable "eth".

- **Fragrance/"Parfum"** – A catchall for unknown chemicals like phthalates. Fragrance has been proven to cause dizziness, headaches, asthma, and even allergic reactions in some unsuspecting victims.

- **Formaldehyde** – A proven irritant and likely carcinogen that can be found in hair dye, nail products, and shampoos. It is already banned in the EU.

- **Lead** – A carcinogenic contaminant found in most lipsticks and hair dyes. Since it's not officially considered to be an ingredient, you'll never see this listed on any beauty product.

- **Hydroquinone** – An ingredient used to peal and lighten skin. It is banned in the UK due to the fact it's been linked to cancer and reproductive disorders.

- **Mineral oil** – This petroleum byproduct can be found in moisturizers, baby oils, and styling gels.

- **Mercury** – An allergen that is known to impair brain function and development. Can be found in select eye drops and mascaras.

- **Parabens** – Used to preserve ingredients in many beauty and baby products. Has been linked to cancer, reproductive disorders, and endocrine problems.

- **Oxybenzone** – A chemical sunscreen that accumulates in fat cells. It can cause allergic reactions and hormone irregularity.

- **Phthalates** – A type of plasticizer that is banned in the EU and just recently, in California. It can be found in perfumes, deodorants, and lotions; and has been linked to kidney, liver, and lung damage.

- **Paraphenylenediamine (PPD)** – Present in hair dyes and styling products. Proven to be toxic to skin and can cause complications with the immune system.

- **Silicone derived emollients** – An ingredient added to some cosmetic products to make them feel soft. It has been linked to skin irritation and tumor enlargement.

- **Talc** – Has a similar composition to asbestos. Can be found in some blushes, eye shadows, baby powders, and deodorants. Has been linked to respiratory problems and ovarian cancer.

- **Sodium lauryl (ether) sulphate (SLS, SLES)** – An ingredient added to soap to make it foamy. It's easily absorbed by the body and can lead to irritation of sensitive skin.

- **Triclosan** – Can be found in some hand sanitizers, deodorants, and antibacterial products. It has been linked to endocrine disorders and cancer.

- **Toluene** – Has been linked to endocrine and

immune disorders. Often found in hair and nail products, this ingredient is often hidden under the term, "fragrance."

Check out the rest of "Homemade Makeup: A Complete Beginner's Guide To Natural DIY Cosmetics You Can Make Today" by Jane Aniston on Amazon.

Check Out My Other Books!

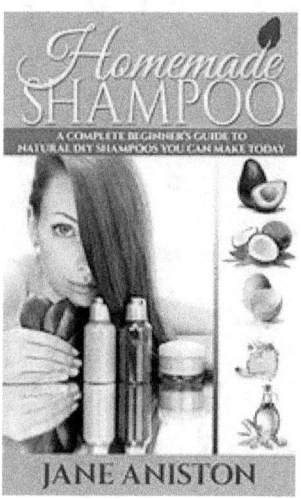

Homemade Shampoo (Includes 34 Organic Shampoo Recipes!)

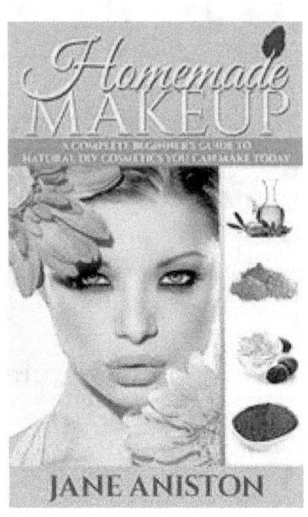

Homemade Makeup (Includes 28 Organic Makeup Recipes!)

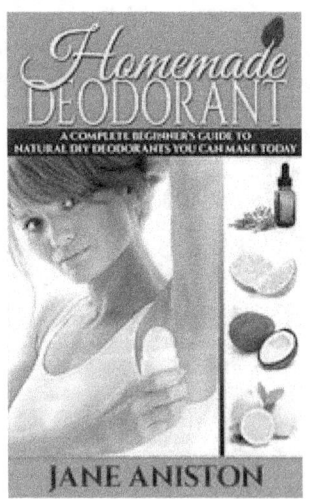

Homemade Deodorant (Includes 20 Organic Deodorant Recipes!)

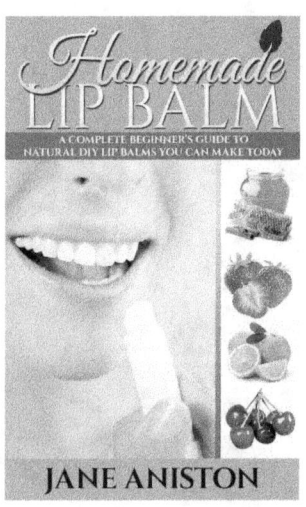

Homemade Lip Balm (Includes 22 Organic Lip Balm Recipes!)

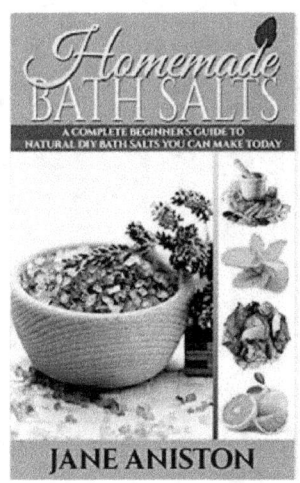

Homemade Bath Salts (Includes 35 Organic Bath Salt Recipes!)